HOME LIFE MEMORIES

A Therapeutic Colouring & Activity Book for Older Adults

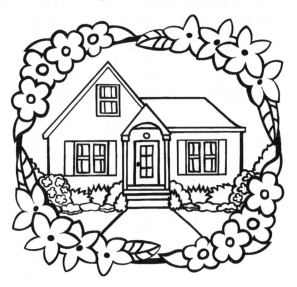

ISBN: 978-0-9951866-0-6

Published by

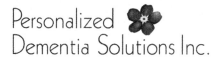
Personalized
Dementia Solutions Inc.

Personalized Dementia Solutions Inc.
www.DementiaSolutions.ca
www.facebook.com/Personalized.Dementia.Solutions.Inc
Twitter: @Dementia_ _Help
Author: Karen Tyrell, CPD, CPCA - www.DementiaSolutions.ca
Illustration and layout: Rose Kapp, www.rosekapp.com
Copy editing team: Hagit Rotbart, BSc, Lisa Kamerling, Gulnar Patel, Bonnie Wannamaker

To order more copies of this book, please visit www.DementiaSolutions.ca

HOME LIFE MEMORIES

A Therapeutic Colouring & Activity Book for Older Adults

This book is a unique engagement tool designed for working one-on-one with older adults to stimulate conversations and preserve memories. It consists of a variety of illustrations and content about familiar items from the 1940s to 1960s and has been created to appeal to the interests of both men and women.

Studies show that Reminiscing Therapy - the main focus of this book - appears to have positive and lasting benefits for older adults, including those affected by mild/moderate dementia. Reminiscing helps to:

- Reduce boredom
- Build closeness in relationships
- Spark stimulating conversations
- Enhance cognitive function

- Improve recollection of past memories
- Lower depression
- Create a fun way to connect with others
- Improve overall mood & quality of life

About this book and how to use it

This therapeutic book is meant to be used for families as well as professional caregivers and recreation professionals as a conversation starter to capture past memories and generate smiles together. Please read out loud and if required, verbally translate or clarify the questions.

Colouring: Provide colouring pencils, crayons or markers that are easy to grip for the older adult you are visiting. Limit the colours if too many choices would cause anxiety or confusion. Tear out the colouring page if you feel it will help with focus, but note that the back of the page may have reminiscing questions for the next illustration.
You can reattach it by using clear plastic tape. A special creative drawing and colouring opportunity has been provided on page 25.

Reminiscing: The colouring illustration on each spread provides a visual, while the corresponding questions on the left are designed to encourage engaging conversations. Sitting on the left side of the older adult who is colouring may help you to read out the reminiscing questions more easily.

Singing: Well-known songs are included throughout the book, to help prompt happy memories. Read out loud or sing the verse and observe the reaction of the person you're visiting.

Cognitive Exercises: This book also assists with cognitive stimulation through exercises ranging from easy to more difficult depending on a person's abilities. These activities can be used over and over again if the answers are done in pencil.

Once all pages are complete, you can tear out the coloured pages and post them as art work on a wall, retain them as a keepsake, or even gift them to a family member or friend. Enjoy!!!

Memories by the Fireplace

1. Tell me about a happy memory you have around a fireplace.

2. Share a story of a time when you used a fireplace to warm yourself.

3. Tell me about a time when you shared a fireplace with a pet who loved it as much as you.

4. What would you do while spending time near a fireplace? (Examples: watch the wood burn, listen to music, socialize, rest, read.)

Some people have warm memories of cuddling by the fireplace with their sweetheart. Do you recall this song?

By The Light of The Silvery Moon
(music by Gus Edwards, lyrics by Edward Madden, 1909)

By the light of the silvery moon
I want to spoon
To my honey, I'll croon love's tune
Honey moon, keep a-shinin' in June
Your silvery beams will bring love's dreams
We'll be cuddlin' soon
By the silvery moon

Another song that may come to mind is "Chestnuts Roasting on an Open Fire" (written by Bob Wells and Mel Tormé, 1945).

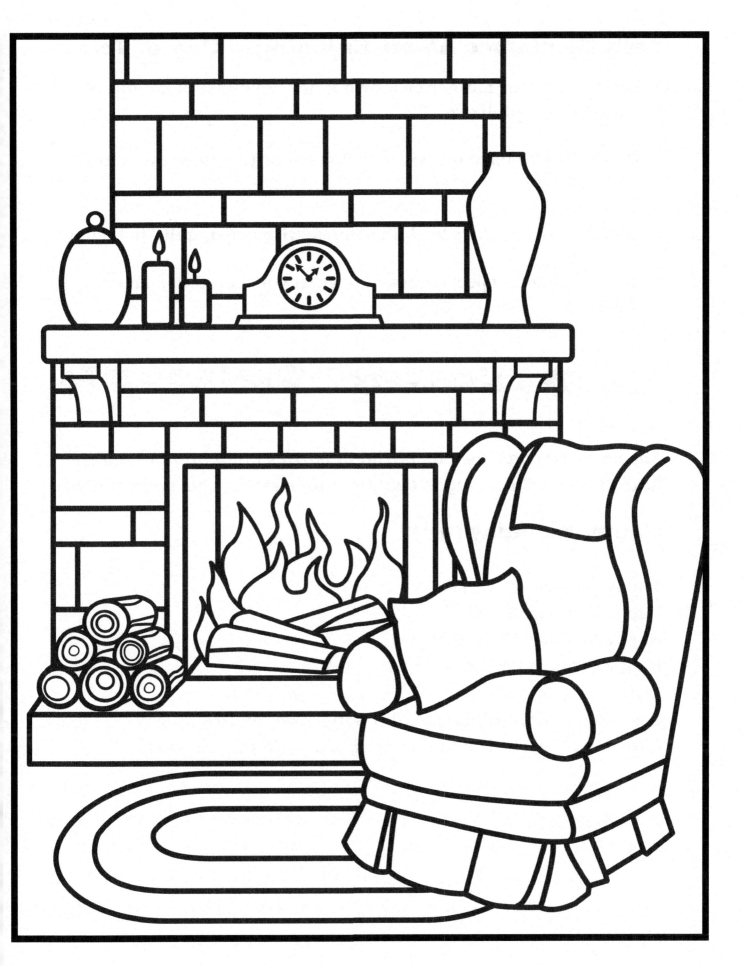

Let's Reminisce About Enjoying a Cup of Tea

1. Did you or your mother ever own fancy tea cups? What did your favourite one look like?

2. Do you prefer tea cups with big flowers or tiny flowers, or any other patterns?

3. How do you like your tea? (Examples: with sugar, milk, hot, cold.)

4. Tell me about a special occasion when you would use fancy teacups.

Special occasions such as birthday parties often brought out the fancy tea set. This song is traditionally sung on this special day.

Happy Birthday (1893)

Happy Birthday to You
Happy Birthday to You
Happy Birthday Dear (name)
Happy Birthday to You

You may also recall the popular song "Tea for Two"
(music by Vincent Youmans and lyrics by Irving Caesar).

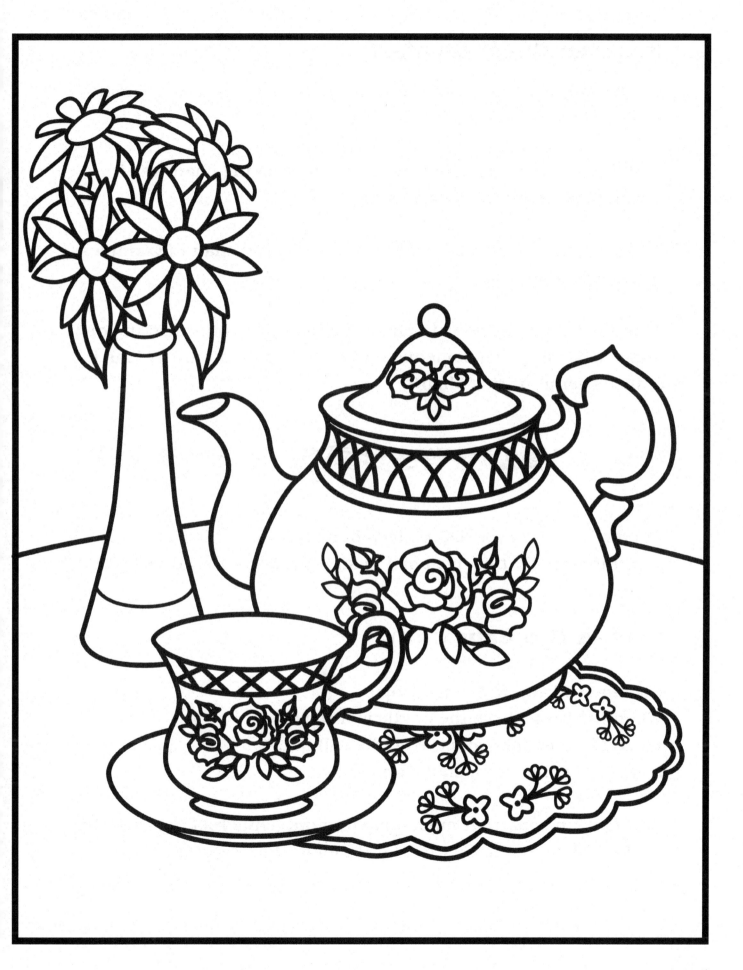

Rocking Chair Comfort

1. What do you remember about the rocking chair in your home and what did it look like?

2. Tell me something about the room the rocking chair was in. (Examples: bedroom; living room.)

3. What did you do when you were in a rocking chair? (Examples: rest, read, rock a baby to sleep.)

4. Tell me about a favourite blanket or quilt you once had in your home. (Example: Did someone make it? Was it colourful? Was it draped over a rocking chair?)

Babies love to be rocked to sleep in a rocking chair. Here's an old popular song that people used to sing while rocking a baby to sleep.

Rock-A-Bye Baby (1872)

Rock-a-bye baby, in the tree top,
When the wind blows the cradle will rock,
When the bough breaks the cradle will fall,
Down will come baby, cradle and all.

Another fun song that may come to mind while rocking in a chair is "Rock Around the Clock" (Bill Haley & His Comets, 1954).

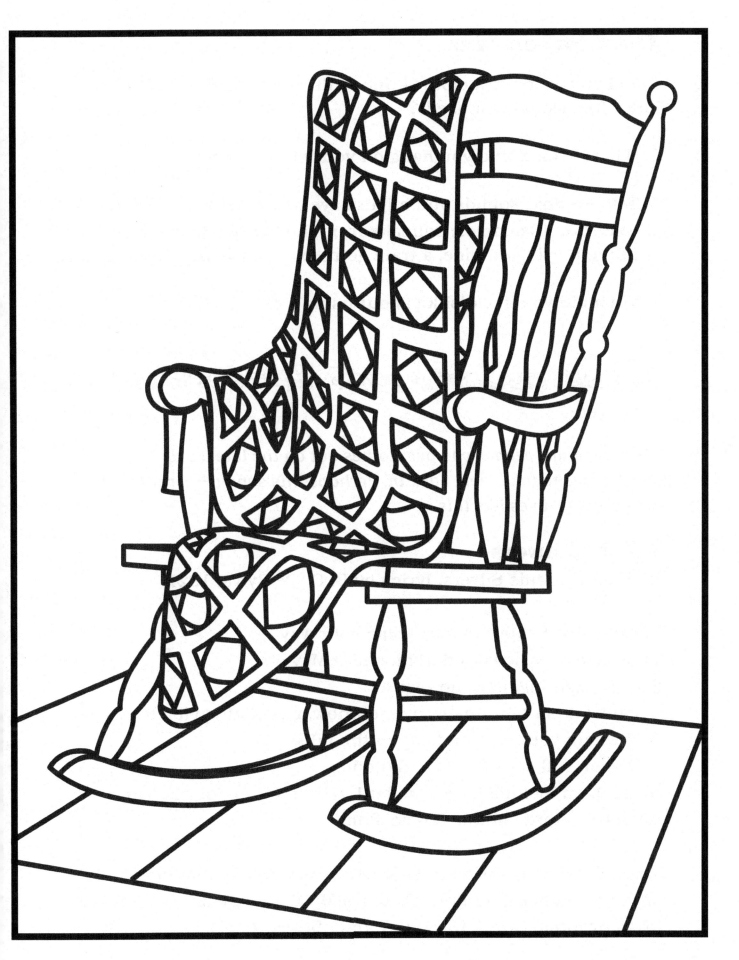

The Clothes Line

1. Did you ever use a clothes line to dry your clothes and, if so, how often would you use it?

2. What items would you hang on your clothes line?

3. Tell me what sounds you might have heard while putting the clothes out. (Examples: squeaks from the clothes line wheel, children playing outside, a train going by, dogs barking.)

4. What did you like/dislike about using a clothes line?

On rainy days, people who put clothes out on the line would have to scramble to take them back in. Perhaps this song will bring back memories of times like this.

April Showers
(written by Louis Silvers, lyrics by B. G. De Sylva, 1921)

Though April showers may come your way
They bring the flowers that bloom in May
So if it's raining, have no regrets
Because it isn't raining rain, you know, it's raining violets
And where you see clouds upon the hills
You soon will see crowds of daffodils
So keep on looking for a blue bird, And list'ning for his song
Whenever April showers come along

When you were putting the clothes on the line while the sun was shining, did you ever sing, "You Are My Sunshine"?
(Rice Brothers Gang, 1939 & Jimmie Davis, 1940).

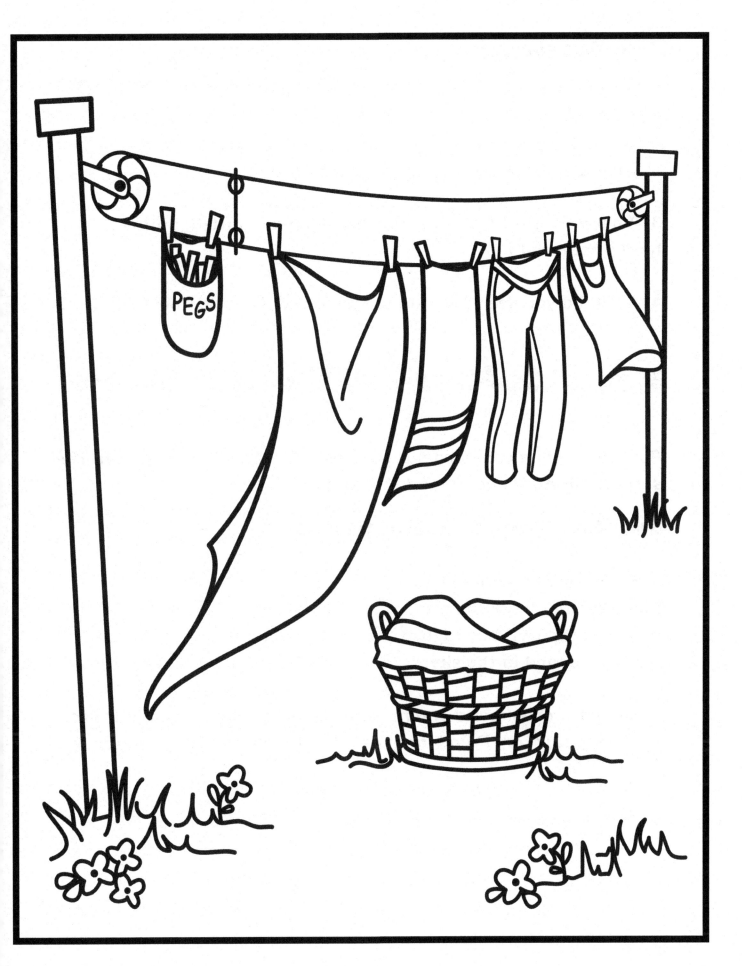

The Bedroom

1. Did you ever share your bedroom with a sibling? If so, how did you like it?

2. What special items were kept in your room?

3. What were your blankets like? (Examples: knitted, quilted, heavy, colourful.)

4. What did you see when you looked out of your bedroom window?

Perhaps you have looked out your bedroom window to gaze at the stars at night. Do you recall this song?

Twinkle, Twinkle Little Star (1806)

Twinkle, twinkle, little star,
How I wonder what you are!
Up above the world so high,
Like a diamond in the sky!

Some may remember a catchy song about waking up called "Are You Sleeping?" or "Frère Jacques" (1780) as it is called in French.

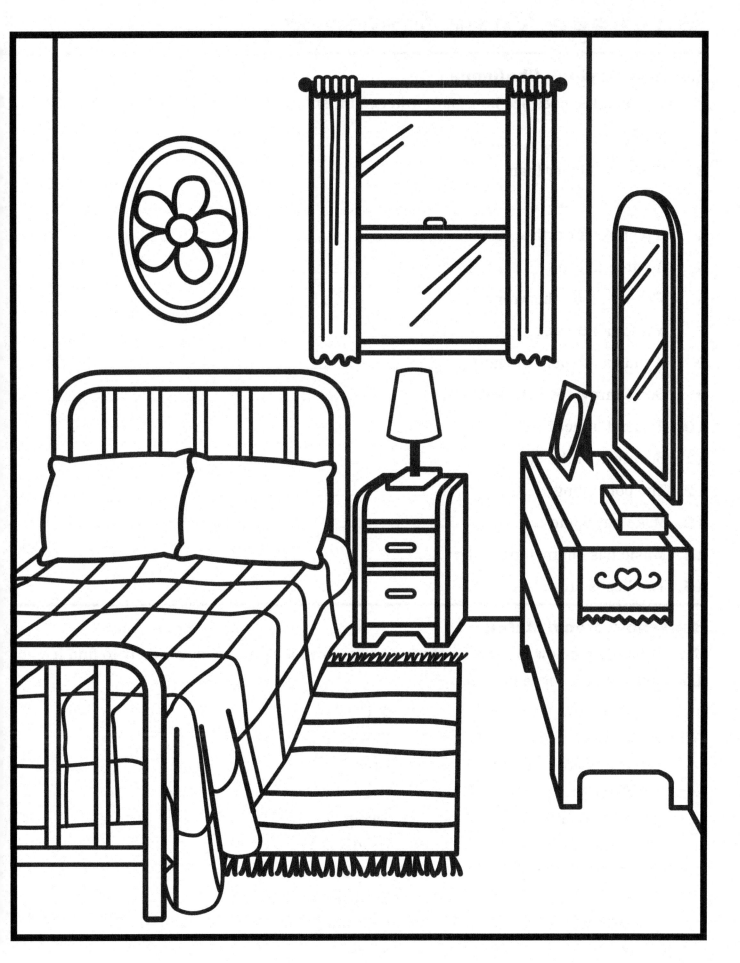

Massage Your Memory (all answers are found on page 26)

Familiar Sayings Challenge

Fill in the blanks. Let's see how many you can finish!

1. Kettle of _____ .

2. Blood is thicker than _____ .

3. Show your true _____ .

4. A picture is worth a _____ _____ .

5. A stitch in time _____ _____ .

6. Waking up on the wrong _____ _____ _____ _____ .

7. Not for all the tea _____ _____ .

8. If you can't stand the heat, _____ _____ _____ _____ _____ .

9. Don't throw the baby out _____ _____ _____ _____ .

10. A friend in need _____ _____ _____ _____ .

11. Beauty is in the eye _____ _____ _____ .

12. The pot calling _____ _____ _____ .

13. Make hay while _____ _____ _____ .

14. Music has charms to soothe _____ _____ _____ .

15. Two heads are _____ _____ _____ .

Household Items Match

Match each item below to the area of your house in which you are most likely to find it. (Use only one area for each item.)

Bedroom	Tub
Closet	Garden rake
Cupboard	Dress
Kitchen	Car
Bathroom	Swing
Entrance	Headboard
Basement	Tea cup
Yard	Storage container
Driveway	Coat hook
Porch	Stove

Massage Your Memory (all answers are found on page 26)

Home Life Trivia Fun

1. What instrument was used to wash clothes before the electric washing machine was invented?

2. Lucille Ball is best known for her role as a wacky housewife on what TV show?

3. What product did Proctor and Gamble launch in 1961 that revolutionized baby care?

4. What was the name of a well-known TV show (1969-1974) about a large, blended family?

5. What household appliance was invented in the late 1960s to cut the overall time needed to prepare meals?

6. What common 1950s laundry detergent claimed to create "the cleanest clean under the sun"?

7. The modern telephone resulted due to the innovative work of many people. Who has most often been credited as the inventor of the first practical telephone?

8. Which movie character advised children that "a spoonful of sugar helps the medicine go down"?

9. In the 1950s, 24% of families owned this household item. Then by 1960, 90% did. What is this item?

10. During the 1960s and 1970s, what did most people in urban environments stop using because of indoor plumbing?

Word Scramble Tease Unscramble these words that all relate to daily life at home.
(Hint: The first letter in questions 1 to 5 is already in the correct spot.)

1. mpo _____

2. lapm _____

3. plilwo _____

4. tebla _____

5. clsote _____

6. rgaedn _____

7. hsdies _____

8. ookbeshfl _____

9. gnironi oradb _____

10. trfegoirraer _____

The Bathroom

1. What did the bathroom look like in one of your past homes?

2. What memories do you have about sharing the bathroom in your house?

3. What did the walls look like in your past bathrooms? (Examples: floral wall paper, tiles, a large mirror, a window.)

4. Do you remember ever using an outhouse where you lived, or perhaps at a cabin? Tell me about it.

Do you recall this funny nursery rhyme about three men in a tub?

Rub-A-Dub-Dub (1789)

Rub-a-dub-dub
Three men in a tub
And who do you think they be?
The butcher, the baker
The candlestick-maker
All put out to sea.

After a great night's sleep, do you ever feel like singing this well-known morning song while freshening up in the bathroom before you start your day? It's called "Oh, What a Beautiful Mornin' " (written by composer Richard Rodgers and lyricist/librettist Oscar Hammerstein II, 1943).

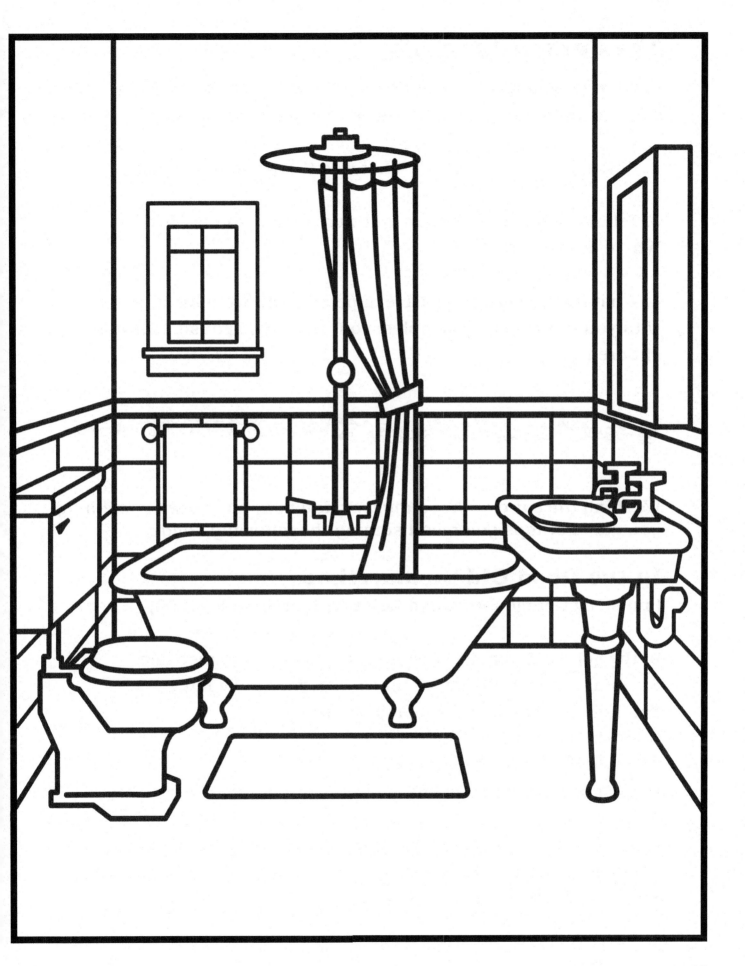

The Cars in Your Life

1. What do you recall about the family car that was used when you were growing up? (Examples: make, model, colour.)

2. Who taught you to drive? What was that experience like?

3. Tell me about a time when you were on a country drive. Where did you often go?

4. What memories do you have of people who were usually with you in the car? (Examples: your parents, spouse, friends, children.)

Washing the car on a hot summer's day may have been something you did. Perhaps you recall singing the following song?

In the Good Old Summertime
(music by George Evans and lyrics by Ren Shields, 1902)

In the good old summertime, in the good old summertime
Strolling through the shady lanes with your baby mine
You hold her hand, and she holds yours
And that's a very good sign
That she's your tootsie-wootsie
in the good old summertime.

Another song some people may remember about cars in the 1960s is a fun tune by the Beach Boys called, "We'll Have Fun, Fun, Fun Till Her Daddy Takes the T'Bird Away" (1964).

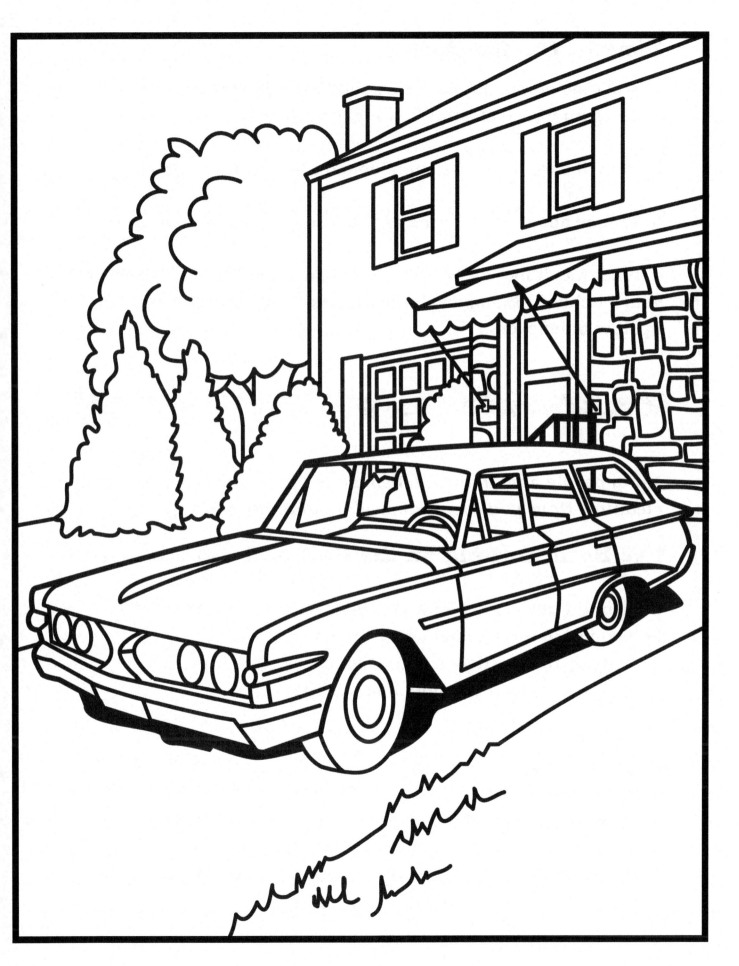

Time in the Kitchen

1. What memories do you have about your kitchen? (Examples: family gatherings, cleaning, eating, cooking.)

2. Describe what your kitchen looked like in a past home.

3. Tell me about some of the appliances you had in your kitchen.

4. What was it like for you after you had a family get-together in your kitchen? (Examples: bit of a mess, many people help clean up, lots of leftovers.)

Many people hum in the kitchen while baking, cooking or cleaning. Have you ever hummed or sung this song?

I've Been Working on the Railroad - second verse (1894)

Someone's in the kitchen with Dinah,
Someone's in the kitchen I know,
Someone's in the kitchen with Dinah,
Strumming on the old banjo, and singing

Fie, fi, fiddly Io,
Fie, fi, fiddly Io,
Fie, fi, fiddly Io,
Strumming on the old banjo.

Perhaps while baking you may have spoken this rhyme –
"Pat-a-Cake, Pat-a-Cake, Baker's Man" (1698).

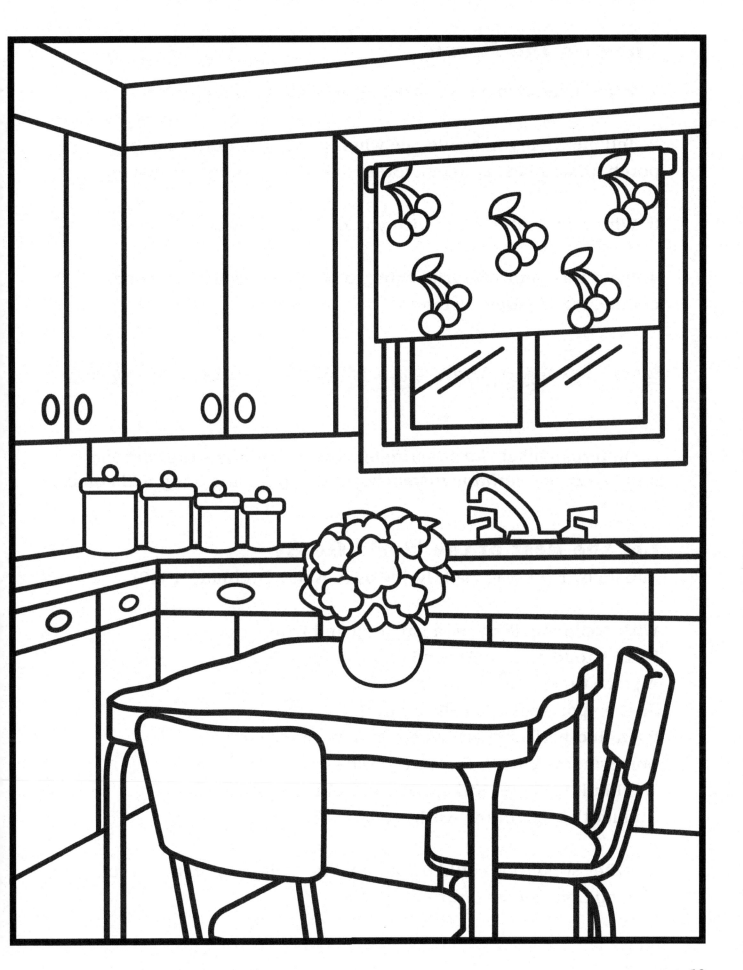

Time on the Porch

1. What memories do you have about sitting on a porch?

2. Tell me what you would see when you gazed out from your porch. (Examples: sunsets, forest, farmland, street, meadow.)

3. Who would sit outside with you on warm summer nights?

4. What was your favourite thing to do on a porch? (Examples: cuddle, read, people watch.)

Do you remember the serenity of warm evenings watching the sun go down? Perhaps memories of the following song will come to mind.

Let the Rest of the World Go By
(music by Ernest R. Ball, lyrics by J. Keirn Brennan, 1919)

With someone like you, a pal good and true,
I'd like to leave it all behind and go and find,
A place that's known to God alone,
Just a spot we could call our own,
We'll find perfect peace where joys never cease,
Somewhere beneath the starry skies,
We'll build a sweet little nest somewhere in the west,
And let the rest of the world go by.

Another song that could be sung while swinging on the porch is "Swing Low, Sweet Chariot" (1909).

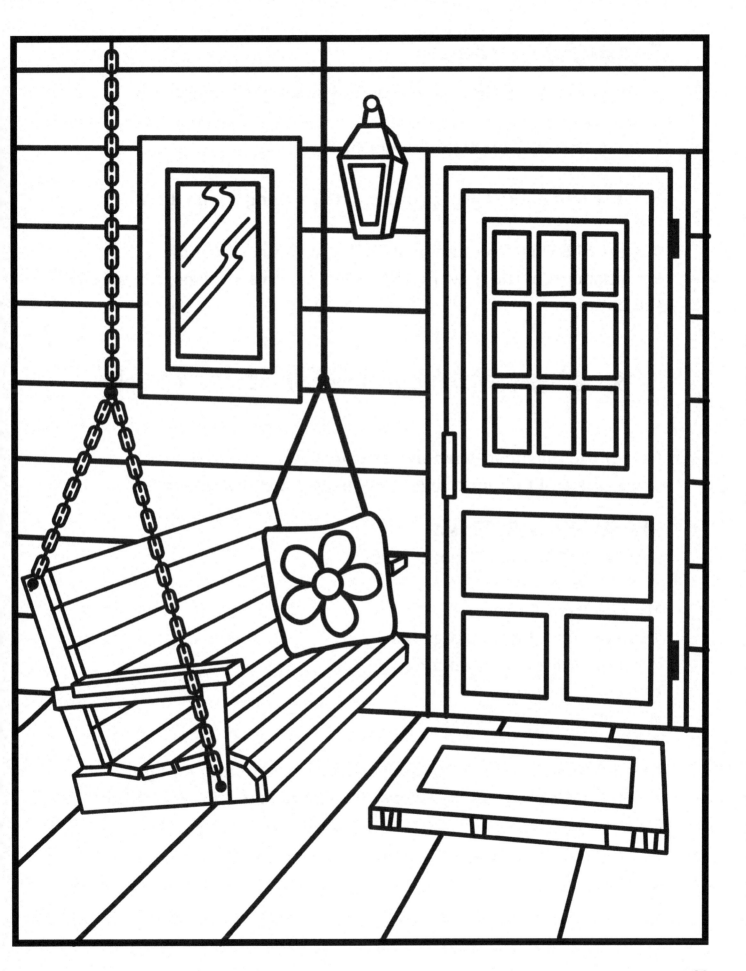

Beautiful Gardens

1. Tell me about a time when you did some gardening.

2. What seeds or plants did you grow?

3. What was it like having your hands working in the dirt?

4. Describe what you like best about gardens. (Examples: the arrangement of the flowers, the taste of the vegetables, the smells, the colours.)

One of the loveliest flowers in the garden is the rose.
Does this song about a wild rose bring back memories?

My Wild Irish Rose
(lyrics by Chauncey Olcott, 1899)

My wild Irish Rose
The sweetest flow'r that grows
You may search ev'rywhere
But none can compare
With my wild Irish Rose.

Another popular hit song about gardens was sung by Lynn Anderson. It was called "I Never Promised You A Rose Garden" (1970).

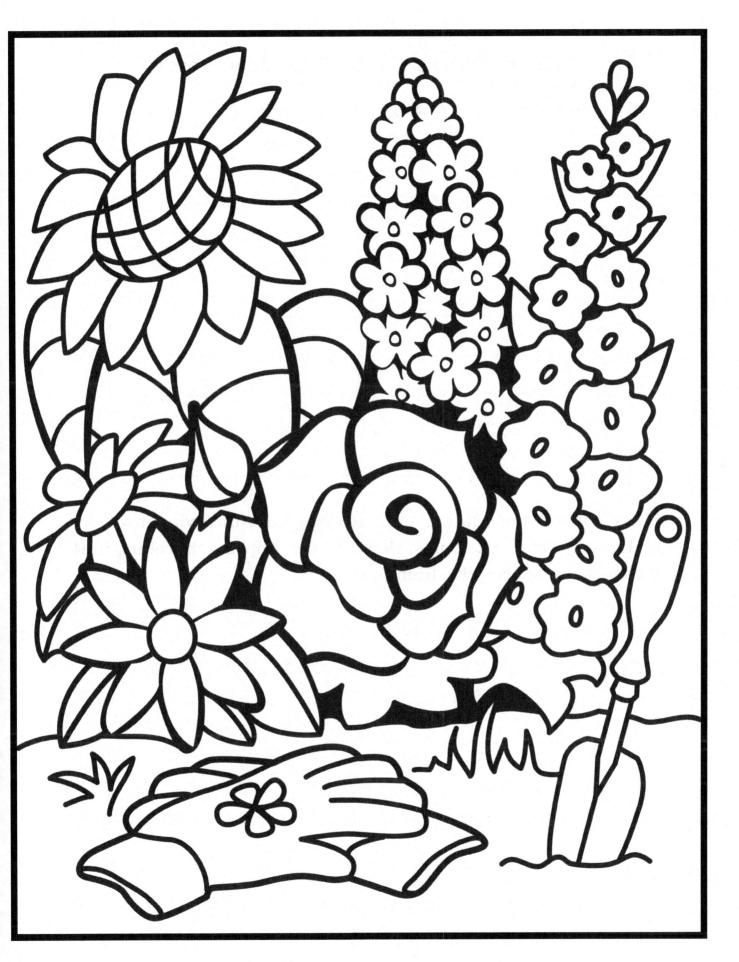

Record Your Home Life Memories

Share a fun home life memory from your past.

_____

_____

_____

_____

_____

_____

Share some of the outdoor activities you did while living in your childhood home. (Examples: riding a bike, hopscotch, rolling in the grass/leaves, sports with friends.)

_____

_____

_____

_____

_____

_____

Now it's your turn...

Try drawing the front of the house where you grew up.
Feel free to colour it in.

Familiar Sayings Challenge

1. Kettle of fish.
2. Blood is thicker than water.
3. Show your true colours.
4. A picture is worth a thousand words.
5. A stitch in time saves nine.
6. Waking up on the wrong side of the bed.
7. Not for all the tea in China.
8. If you can't stand the heat, stay out of the kitchen.
9. Don't throw the baby out with the bathwater.
10. A friend in need is a friend indeed.
11. Beauty is in the eye of the beholder.
12. The pot calling the kettle black.
13. Make hay while the sun shines.
14. Music has charms to soothe the savage beast.
15. Two heads are better than one.

Home Life Trivia Fun

1. A washboard
2. I Love Lucy
3. Disposable diapers
4. The Brady Bunch
5. The microwave oven
6. Tide
7. Alexander Graham Bell
8. Mary Poppins
9. Television
10. The outhouse

Household Items Match

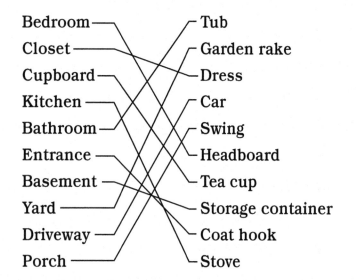

Bedroom — Tub
Closet — Garden rake
Cupboard — Dress
Kitchen — Car
Bathroom — Swing
Entrance — Headboard
Basement — Tea cup
Yard — Storage container
Driveway — Coat hook
Porch — Stove

Word Scramble Tease

1. mop
2. lamp
3. pillow
4. table
5. closet
6. garden
7. dishes
8. bookshelf
9. ironing board
10. refrigerator

"Growing old is mandatory, but growing up is optional."
~ Walt Disney

CPSIA information can be obtained
at www.ICGtesting.com
Printed in the USA
LVOW05s2150030118
561667LV00023B/225/P

9 780995 186606